Paleo Coconut Oil

Miracle

Super Easy, Delicious and Quick Recipes

Contents

About the Book 4

Introduction...5

Breakfast..6

    Paleo Cereal 6

    Date & Chocolate Granola Bars 7

    Strawberry Breakfast Muffins w/ Almonds 9

    Maple & Date Granola 11

    Breakfast Muffins w/ Egg 13

    Plantain Breakfast "Patties" 15

Sweets & Desserts...16

    Chocolate Cake w/ Coffee Frosting.....................16

    Savory Coconut Balls..18

    Chocolate Chip Cookies w/ Macadamia Nuts 19

    Caramel Brownies w/ Cherries 21

    Strawberry Spheres..23

    Vanilla Cheese Cake 24

Sides & Appetizers...25

    Sweet & Spicy Sweet Potato Slices 25

    Sweet Potato Salad 26

    Pineapple Guacamole & Plantain Chips..............28

    Stuffed Sweet Potato Skins 30

    Bison Bites...32

    Sliders..34

    Turkey Meatball Bites 36

Dinner Entrees..38

Coconut Chicken Patties w/ Almonds.................................38

Salmon Patties w/ Parsley..40

Coconut Shrimp..41

Indian Style Chicken & Rice..43

Cherry Chicken 45

Mango Beef w/ Plantain 47

About the Book

This is a book for followers and newcomers to the Paleolithic diet. Learn the guidelines of the diet in the introduction. Then get inspired to try out new dishes, which follow the diet guidelines, in a collection of recipes. This book specializes with the ingredient of coconut oil. Coconut oil has health benefits of its own in addition to the Paleo diet's benefits. The recipes in this book start out with breakfast dishes, then continue to sweets and desserts, sides and appetizers and lastly dinner entrees. Enjoy cooking your way to health by trying out these healthy and delicious ideas.

Introduction

Paleolithic eating is a diet made up of wild plant and animal foods. The diet is what hunter-gatherers ate in the Paleolithic era starting 2.5 million years ago through 10,000 years ago. At that point, the development of agriculture introduced grain-based diets. The theory behind Paleolithic eating believes that humans are not genetically adapted new way of eating composed of processed foods, high refined carbohydrates and wheat. Paleo is composed of meats, seafood, fresh fruits and vegetables.

The guidelines of the diet include 60% animal sources and 40% plant sources. Excluded are cereal grains, legumes, dairy, refined sugar, processed foods, salt and refined vegetable oils. The framework includes higher intake of protein, fiber, potassium, omega 6 and 3 polyunsaturated/ monounsaturated fats, alkaline foods, vitamins, minerals, antioxidants and plant phytochemicals. By eliminating foods, the diet lowers carbohydrate intake, glycemic index, and sodium. Consuming this diet has shown to reduce health problems such as weight gain, cardiovascular disease, diabetes, metabolic syndrome, and gastrointestinal tract diseases, to name a few. Going back to these basics, has shown promise to optimize health, reduce disease and maintain a healthy weight. Enjoy eating your way to a healthier body with these recipes.

Breakfast

Paleo Cereal

Serves 3

3 tbsp. coconut oil (melted)

1¼ c. organic almond flour

3 tbsp. coconut flour

2 tbsp. coconut sugar

1 tbsp. ground cinnamon

¼ tsp. sea salt

1 egg white

1/3 c. raw honey

Heat up the oven to 350 and line a baking sheet with parchment paper. You will need two mixing bowls. In the first one combine the flours, sugar, salt and cinnamon. In the second bowl, beat the egg white and combine the melted oil and honey. Slowly mix the flour mixture into the egg mixture. Mix thoroughly and then roll the dough into small puffs. Bake 15 minutes and let cool. Store in an air tight container.

Date & Chocolate Granola Bars

Serves 10

4 tbsp. melted coconut oil

1 c. chopped and roasted almonds

½ c. chopped and roasted macadamia nuts

½ c. shredded coconut (unsweetened)

5 tbsp. unsweetened cocoa powder

¼ c. cherries (dried)

6 Pitted and diced dates

2 tbsp. raw honey

¼ tsp. sea salt

Heat up the oven to 320 and line a baking sheet with parchment paper. Combine the nuts, salt and cocoa together in the food processor. Process the ingredients until they are chopped and well combined. Then pour the mixture into a mixing bowl with the coconut, dates and cherries. Mix well. In a saucepan, melt the coconut oil over medium heat and then add honey and melt. Mix the honey oil into the nuts mixture and sprinkle on the parchment paper. Place another sheet of parchment paper on top and press down. Take the top piece off and bake 15 minutes.

Cool and store in the fridge. Then cut into rectangles. Store in an airtight container.

Strawberry Breakfast Muffins w/ Almonds

Serves 12

¼ c. melted coconut oil

2 c. sifted almond flour

1½ tsp. baking soda

¼ tsp. sea salt

4 large eggs

1 tbsp. vanilla (extract)

8 pitted dates

1¼ c. fresh sliced strawberries

Crumble Topping:

1 tbsp. melted coconut oil

1/3 c. chopped macadamia nuts

1/3 c. chopped walnuts

2 tbsp. raw coconut sugar

Heat up the oven to 350 and line a muffin pan w2ith cupcake liners. Make the crumbles first by combining the coconut oil, chopped nuts, chopped walnuts and sugar until well combined. Set aside. Now for the muffins, combine the baking soda, salt and flour until well combined. Puree the wet ingredients in the food processor until completely combined. Slowly mix them into the flour bowl and beat until batter is smooth. Then add in the strawberries. Divide the batter between the muffin cups and top with the crumble. Bake 25 minutes then let cool.

Maple & Date Granola

16 Servings

2/3 c. melted coconut oil

1 c. pumpkin seeds

2/3 c. shredded coconut (unsweetened)

1 c. almonds (thin sliced)

1 c. pecans (chopped)

20 diced and pitted dates

1 c. fresh pumpkin puree

2/3 c. raw maple syrup

2 tsp. vanilla extract

2 tbsp. ground nutmeg

2 tbsp. ground cinnamon

¼ tsp. all-spice

¼ tsp. ground ginger

¼ tsp. sea salt

Heat up the oven to 320 and prepare baking sheets with parchment paper. In a mixing bowl mix together the nuts, seeds, coconut, spices and salt. Mix well. In a separate bowl mix the oil, pumpkin, syrup and vanilla until smooth. Mix the pumpkin mix into the nut mixture and stir until thoroughly combined. Then fold the dates into the mixture. Spread the mixture out on the baking sheet and bake for 30 minutes. Stir up the granola after 20 minutes. Let it cool down then be sure to store it in an air tight container.

Breakfast Muffins w/ Egg

36 Servings

1 tbsp. melted coconut oil

1 lb. ground bison (preferably organic)

22 large eggs

½ c. whole coconut milk

1 tbsp. curry

1 small white onion (diced)

5 white mushrooms (thin sliced)

2 carrots (grated)

2 broccoli stems (chopped)

Sea salt to taste

Pepper to taste

Coconut oil spray

Heat up the oven to 375 and line muffin tins with cupcake liners. Melt the coconut oil in a large skillet over medium heat. Sauté the onions until they soften and season with salt and pepper. Once softened, add the salt and pepper to taste. Next, brown the meat and sprinkle curry powder on it. Once browned, add in the chopped broccoli and carrots. Once they soften set that aside away from the heat. In a large bowl, crack all the eggs and whisk them until yolks are broken up and well incorporated. Then mix in the milk, salt and pepper. Divide the bison mixture between the muffin cups and top by dividing the egg mixture. Bake 20 minutes then enjoy!

Plantain Breakfast "Patties"

4 Servings

4 tbsp. of coconut oil

2 blackened plantains (peeled and sliced)

Sea salt to taste

1 lime (slice)

Heat up a large skillet and melt the coconut oil. Add the plantains into it and let them lightly brown on one side, then flip them and brown the other side. Then remove from the heat, place on a plate with a paper towel and sprinkle them with sea salt. Flatten each one out and then add them back into the skillet, frying for a minute or two. Then remove them and drain them again. Sprinkle salt and lime juice and serve.

.

Sweets & Desserts

Chocolate Cake w/ Coffee Frosting

10-12 Servings

Cake:

1 tbsp. melted coconut oil

2 sweet potatoes (baked)

1 tbsp. sifted coconut flour

8 oz. raw chocolate (unsweetened)

¼ c. raw cacao powder (unsweetened)

¼ c. raw honey

3 large eggs

1 tsp. vanilla extract

1 tsp. baking soda

½ tsp. sea salt

Coconut oil (spray)

Frosting:

1 c. melted coconut oil

1½ tsp. vanilla extract

3 tbsp. whole coconut milk

1 tbsp. coconut crystals

¼ c. fresh coconut (shredded)

4 oz. fine coffee grounds

Cake:

Heat up the oven to 325 and grease a baking sheet with coconut oil. Process the sweet potatoes until smooth then mix in remaining ingredients. When smooth, transfer the mix into a baking dish. Bake 40 minutes then remove. Refrigerate for about 5 hours.

.Frosting:

Beat the coconut oil rapidly for about 5 minutes until it becomes fluffy. Then add in and process the coconut crystals, milk and vanilla and mix thoroughly. Mix in the coconut and coffee grounds. Spread on the cake and enjoy!

Savory Coconut Balls

15 Servings

5 tbsp. melted coconut oil

3 cups unsweetened shredded coconut

2 tsp. vanilla extract

3/8 tsp. sea salt

Like a baking sheet with parchment paper. Combine the ingredients together in a food processor and pulse for about 5 minutes or until moist and well combined. Then roll the mixture into balls the size of about 2 tbsp. Line them up on the parchment paper and chill for an hour in the fridge.

Chocolate Chip Cookies w/ Macadamia Nuts

20 Servings

½ c. melted coconut oil

2½ c. sifted almond flour

2 tbsp. sifted coconut flour

2/3 c. shredded coconut (unsweetened)

1 tsp. baking soda

¼ c. raw honey

3 large eggs (whisked)

1 tbsp. vanilla extract

2/3 c. chopped macadamia nuts (roasted)

2/3 c. chocolate chips (unsweetened)

¼ tsp. sea salt

Heat up the oven to 350 and line baking sheets with foil. In a large bowl mic the flours, coconut, salt and baking soda together thoroughly. In another bowl, beat the eggs until frothy and mix with vanilla, honey and oil. Slowly mix the egg mixture into the flour bowl and combine well. Once your batter is smooth, add in the nuts and chocolate until well combined. Scoop out dough (about 2 tbsp. each) and place them into flattened circles on the foil. Bake about 20 minutes.

Caramel Brownies w/ Cherries

9 Servings

1/3 c. melted coconut oil

2½ c. sifted almond flour

¼ c. cocoa powder (unsweetened)

1 tsp. baking soda

¼ tsp. sea salt

2 large eggs

½ c. raw maple syrup

½ c. chopped macadamia nuts (roasted and unsalted)

½ c. dark chocolate chips

¼ c. dried cherries

½ c. toasted coconut flakes (unsweetened)

Heat up the oven to 350 and grease a baking dish. Combine the flour, salt, baking soda and cocoa together and combine thoroughly. In another bowl, beat the eggs until frothy and add the syrup and oil and mix well. Then stir the egg mixture into the flour mixture and combine until smooth. Once smooth, fold in the nuts, cherries and chocolate chips. Transfer into the baking dish and bake 30 minutes. Let cool, top with toasted coconut and refrigerate for about an hour. Slice and serve.

Strawberry Spheres

10 Servings

3 tbsp. melted coconut oil

1 c. chopped walnuts

¾ c. chopped macadamia nuts (roasted)

5 pitted dates

½ c. diced strawberries

½ c. shredded coconut (unsweetened)

Prepare a baking sheet by lining it with parchment paper. Then process the pitted dates in a food processor until they make a paste. Then combine the walnuts and macadamia nuts into the dates and process until fine. Gradually pour in the oil as you are pulsing the processor. Once oil is fully mixed in, add the mixture into a bowl and fold in the diced strawberries. Roll them into balls and cover them in shredded coconut. Then line them on the parchment paper. Refrigerate for 2 hours.

Vanilla Cheese Cake

10 Servings

¾ c. melted coconut oil

1 c. pitted dates

2 c. pecans (halved)

2 c. cashews (soak overnight)

1 tsp. vanilla extract

½ c. lime juice (fresh)

½ c. raw maple syrup

¼ c. water (filtered)

¼ tsp. sea salt

Process the pecans and dates in the food processor until they form a paste like consistency. Then spread it to cover the bottom of a cheesecake pan. Press it down tight. Then in a clean processor, combine the lime juice, water, salt, vanilla, syrup and oil. Process until smooth. Pour this layer on top of the crust. Cover and freeze for 6 hours. Remove from freezer about 30 minutes before eating. Slice

Sides & Appetizers

Sweet & Spicy Sweet Potato Slices

4 Servings

1/3 c. melted coconut oil

2 large sweet potatoes

1 tbsp. ground peppercorns

2 tsp. sage (dried)

1 tbsp. oregano (dried)

1 tbsp. thyme (dried)

2 tbsp. paprika (dried)

1 tsp. ground cayenne pepper

3 tsp. garlic powder

Heat up the grill on medium. In a boiling pot of water, blanch the potatoes for about 5 minutes, then combine all seasonings in one bowl and cover the potatoes in oil then seasoning. Make sure all potatoes are thoroughly covered. Place on the grill for about 10 minutes.

Sweet Potato Salad

3 Servings

2 tbsp. melted coconut oil

1 medium sweet potato (diced)

2 large eggs (hard boiled)

¼ c. white onion (chopped)

Mayo:

⅔ c. avocado oil

1 medium egg

1 tsp. fresh lemon juice

1 tsp. mustard

½ tsp. parsley (dried flakes)

½ tsp. thyme (dried)

½ tsp. basil (dried)

Salt to taste

Pepper to taste

Heat up the oven to 400 and grease a baking sheet. Place the diced tomatoes in a medium bowl and coat them with oil. Transfer to a baking sheet and bake 20 minutes. Cool them off. Meanwhile, boil the eggs. Once hard boiled, peel and chop them. Next make the mayo by combining all the ingredients in an immersion blender. Once combined, mix the cool potatoes, chopped eggs, onion and mayo in a bowl. Season to taste and serve.

Pineapple Guacamole & Plantain Chips

3 Servings

2 tbsp. melted coconut oil

2 avocados (pitted and halved)

½ c. pineapple (diced)

2 green plantains (sliced)

1 blackened plantain (smashed or pureed)

½ c. jalapeno (diced)

¼ Red onion (diced)

3 tbsp. cilantro (chopped)

2 cloves of garlic (diced)

1 tsp. garlic powder

½ tsp. cayenne pepper

Salt to taste

Pepper to taste

Heat the grill up to medium-high. Slice the blackened plantains and coat them in coconut oil. Sprinkle them with salt and grill them for about 10 minutes per side. Meanwhile, melt coconut oil in a large skillet and add sliced green plantains to it. Cook for 5 minutes per side so that they are thoroughly browned. Drain on a paper towel. In a medium bowl, add the avocado flesh and mix it until smooth. Then combine the salt, pepper, onion, jalapeno, pineapple, spices, cilantro and garlic and mix until smooth. Let the chips cool, then dip them in the avocado and pineapple dip.

Stuffed Sweet Potato Skins

5 Servings

2 tbsp. melted coconut oil

3 medium sweet potatoes

½ red onion (diced)

2 avocados (pitted)

½ fresh juiced lime

½ fresh juiced lemon

1 tsp. ground cumin

Salt to taste

Pepper to taste

1 lb. chorizo (casings removed)

1 tbsp. almond flour

Heat up the oven to 425 and prepare a baking sheet with coconut oil. Poke holes in the potatoes with a fork and line them on the baking sheet. Bake 25 minutes until soft. Sauté the chorizo in a large skillet over medium-high heat. When about half way done cooking, add in the onions. Then drain it on a paper towel when finished. Process the flesh of two avocados to a smooth consistency. Once smooth, add in lemon, lime, salt and cumin. Process. Reserve ¼ of the mixture. In a large bowl mix the rest of the avocado mix with the chorizo. Remove the potatoes from the oven and halve them. Scoop the insides out and brush the skin with oil. Bake 15 minutes then remove. Stuff each one with the chorizo mixture and bake 5 more minutes. Top with reserved avocado mixture.

Bison Bites

12 Servings

2 lbs. bison meat (ground)

1 tbsp. melted coconut oil

14 oz. diced tomatoes

6 oz. fresh tomato paste

3 diced garlic cloves

1 diced yellow onion

1 c. water (filtered)

2 tbsp. fresh thyme (chopped)

2 tbsp. ground paprika

4 tsp. ground cumin

2 tsp. sea salt

½ tsp. ground black pepper

¼ c. chopped pistachios (roasted and shelled)

In a small bowl combine the seasonings: salt, pepper, cumin, thyme, and paprika. Mix in the bison. Form the meat into 12 balls. Melt the coconut oil in a large skillet over medium heat. Add onions and let them soften, then add in the garlic along with salt, pepper, cumin and paprika. Then add in tomato paste and the diced tomatoes. Turn up the heat so that it boils. Lower the heat back down and add the meatballs. Cover and simmer for 45 minutes. Remove the lid and simmer another 15 minutes. The sauce should get thicker.

Sliders

4 Servings

1 tbsp. melted coconut oil

1 lb. ground beef

2 tbsp. ground cinnamon

1½ tbsp. powdered garlic

1½ onion powder

1 tsp. chili powder

½ tsp. cayenne pepper

¼ tsp. paprika

Sea salt to taste

Pepper to taste

1 thin sliced red onion

10 mushrooms (thin sliced)

2 Tbsp. balsamic vinegar

2 Tbsp. olive oil (extra virgin)

Mix the beef with the spices in a bowl until thoroughly incorporated. Melt the coconut oil in a large skillet over medium heat. Once heated add the onions and a tbsp. of water. Once browned, increase the heat to medium-high. Make the mat into 3 inch flat rounds and add them to the skillet. Cook 5 minutes, flip then cook another 5 minutes. Keep the onions moving so that they don't get burnt. After about 8 minutes, add the sliced mushrooms and a tbsp. more of water. Lastly, add the vinegar. Serve the sliders topped with the sautéed onions and garlic.

Turkey Meatball Bites

20 Servings

2 lbs. turkey (ground)

2 large eggs

1 small bell pepper (red, chopped)

1 small bell pepper (green, chopped)

½ red onion (chopped)

3 cloves of garlic (finely diced)

¼ c. sifted almond flour

1 tsp. salt

1 tsp. pepper

1 tsp. parsley

Coconut oil

Melt the coconut oil over medium heat in a large skillet. Once heated, add the onions and sauté until softened. Once softened, add the bell pepper until softened. Then add the garlic. Pour all the skillet contents into a mixing bowl. Set aside. In another large bowl, beat the eggs, add salt, pepper, flour, turkey and the skillet mix. Set a piece of parchment paper on a baking sheet and line up meatballs on it. In a clean large skillet, melt coconut oil over medium high. Fry the meatballs for about 5 minutes per side. Add the lid to cook the insides.

Dinner Entrees

Coconut Chicken Patties w/ Almonds

6 Servings

3 Tbsp. melted coconut oil

2 Lb. ground chicken (organic free-range)

2 egg yolks

½ C. sifted almond flour

½ C. shredded coconut (unsweetened)

2 Tsp. onion powder

2 Tsp. garlic powder

½ Tsp. sea salt

½ Tsp. ground pepper

Start by placing all your ingredients minus the coconut oil in a bowl and mixing well. Set a skillet on medium heat and add a tablespoon and a half of coconut oil to melt. When the oil has melted, start to form your chicken patties by hand and placing them in the oil. Cook each patty for five to six minutes, at this point the bottoms should be brown. Remove from the heat and let cool slightly to set before serving.

Salmon Patties w/ Parsley

2-4 Servings

3 Tbsp. melted coconut oil

18 Oz. fresh salmon

½ C. chopped parsley

½ Purple onion (chopped)

1/3 C. sifted almond flour

¼ Tsp. ground pepper

1 Tsp. sea salt

3 Large eggs (beaten)

Start off by thoroughly mixing your salmon and eggs together in a large bowl. In a separate bowl mix up the onions, salt, pepper, parsley, and almond flour and then combine with the first mix. Set a skillet on medium heat and add the coconut oil. Form patties from the salmon and egg mix and fry until crisp. Use a towel to absorb any excess oil from your patties and lightly salt and pepper.

Coconut Shrimp

4 Servings

1 lb. Peeled and uncooked shrimp

1 Tbsp. coconut oil

6 Oz. whole coconut milk

3 Whisked eggs whites

⅓ C. sifted coconut flour

1 C. shredded coconut (unsweetened)

3 Tbsp. curry powder (yellow)

1 Tsp. ground cayenne

½ Tsp. sriracha

½ Tsp. sea salt

½ Tsp. ground pepper

1 Garlic clove (thin sliced)

1 Juiced lime

Begin by whisking your egg whites until they are foamy and peaks begin to form. Then, in a separate bowl, mix two tablespoons of curry powder together with the flour, cayenne, salt and pepper. Next gather a third bowl and pour the shredded coconut in. Gather your shrimp and dip it in the egg bowl, then in the flour bowl and finally in the shredded coconut. Repeat until all the shrimp are coated evenly. Heat your skillet on medium heat and add a little coconut oil and a garlic clove. When warmed add in the coconut milk, curry powder and sriracha and let it simmer down a bit. When the texture becomes thick add in your shrimp and cook thoroughly. Serve warm.

Indian Style Chicken & Rice

4 Servings

2 Tbsp. melted coconut oil

1Lb. chicken breast (cubed)

1 Cauliflower head (stemmed and blended to make "rice")

½ C. whole coconut milk

14 Oz. fresh tomato sauce

½ Diced onion

2 Minced garlic cloves

2 Tbsp. raw honey

1 Juiced lemon

2 Tbsp. curry

2 Tsp. garam marsala

1 Tsp. ground paprika

1 Tsp. ground cinnamon

1 Tsp. ground cumin

½ Tsp. coriander

½ Tsp. ground cloves

½ Tsp. ground ginger

Dash of salt

Dash of pepper

Start by sautéing your garlic and onions in a skillet with the coconut oil until translucent. Once cooked, pour in your coconut milk, lemon juice, honey, spices and tomato paste and mix thoroughly. When simmering, add in your chicken and "rice" and cook for another ten minutes.

Cherry Chicken

4 Servings

1 Lb. chopped chicken thighs

2 Thin sliced shallots

2 Tbsp. melted coconut oil

2 C. fresh cherries (pitted)

⅛ C. red wine vinegar

¼ C. balsamic vinegar

2 Tsp. ground cinnamon

2 Tbsp. dried tarragon

1 Tsp. dried ground ginger

½ Tsp. dried ground oregano

½ Tsp. dried thyme

1 C. thin sliced almonds

Dash of sea salt

Dash of ground pepper

Start by melting a tablespoon of coconut oil in a saucepan on medium heat. When the oil is warm, add in the shallots and cook until translucent. Next turn down the heat to low and stir in your vinegars, cinnamon, tarragon cherries, salt and pepper. Let simmer for about five minutes. You can now start cooking your chicken in a large skillet on medium heat. Add in a tablespoon of coconut oil along with your seasonings and cook thoroughly. Serve this chicken with your cherry sauce and some roasted almonds.

Mango Beef w/ Plantain

4 Servings

12 Oz. sirloin steak (cut to strips)

3 Tbsp. melted coconut oil

1 Sliced yellow onion

2 minced garlic cloves

1 plantain, ends removed, peeled and sliced into ¼ inch pieces, smashed (use a ripe one-brownish color)

1 Cubed mango

2 Tsp. curry powder

1 Tsp. garlic powder

1 Tsp. ground red pepper

¼ Tsp. sea salt

¼ Tsp. ground pepper

Start by heating a skillet on medium heat; add in your garlic and a tablespoon of coconut oil with the sliced onions. Allow those to cook while you while you fry your plantains in an additional skillet on high heat. Now while your plantains are cooking, add in the sirloin to the skillet with your onions in it. When the sirloin is about done cooking, stir in the powdered garlic, salt, pepper, ground red pepper and mango. Cook for an additional two minutes and then remove from heat and gently stir in your fried plantains. Allow to cool slightly and serve.

www.ingramcontent.com/pod-product-compliance
Lightning Source LLC
Chambersburg PA
CBHW070230290526
45789CB00004B/1569